All About BREAST CANCER | ELI TOBY

TABLE OF CONTENT

<u>Foreword:</u>

Breast cancer is a significant health concern for women worldwide. It is the most common cancer among women, and early detection and treatment are essential for improving outcomes. In this book, we will explore the science behind breast cancer, its different types, causes, risk factors, symptoms, diagnosis, and treatment options. We will also discuss the emotional and psychological impact of breast cancer on patients and their loved ones, as well as strategies for coping and living with breast cancer.

<u>Chapter 1.</u>

Understanding Breast Cancer.

In this chapter, we will define what breast cancer is, how it develops, and the different stages of breast cancer. We will also explain the various types of breast cancer and how they differ from one another. We will discuss the role of genetics and environmental factors in the development of breast cancer.

Breast cancer is a type of cancer that forms in the cells of the breast. It is the most common cancer in women, but it can also occur in men. Breast cancer usually begins as a small, painless lump in the breast, but it can also cause other symptoms such as changes in the size or shape of the breast, dimpling or puckering of the skin, nipple discharge, or redness or thickening of the skin of the breast or nipple.

*How does breast cancer develop?

Breast cancer develops when the cells in the breast begin to grow and divide uncontrollably, forming a lump or mass. These cancer cells can invade nearby tissues and spread to other parts of the body, such as the lymph nodes or distant organs, through the bloodstream or lymphatic system.

*The different stages of breast cancer.

Breast cancer is staged based on the size of the tumor, whether it has spread to nearby lymph nodes, and whether it has spread to other parts of the body. The most commonly used staging system for breast cancer is the TNM system, which stands for Tumor, Node, Metastasis.

Here are the stages of breast cancer according to the TNM system:

Stage 0: This is called ductal carcinoma in situ (DCIS). The cancer cells are contained within the milk ducts and have not spread to nearby tissue.

Stage I: The tumor is small, usually less than 2 cm, and has not spread to nearby lymph nodes or other parts of the body.

Stage II: The tumor is larger, usually between 2-5 cm, and may or may not have spread to nearby lymph nodes.

Stage III: The tumor is larger and has spread to nearby lymph nodes or other nearby tissue, but has not spread to distant organs.

Stage IV: The cancer has spread to distant organs, such as the bones, lungs, or liver. This is also called metastatic breast cancer.

The stage of breast cancer is an important factor in determining the best course of treatment. Early-stage breast cancer is often treated with surgery to remove the tumor, followed by radiation therapy, chemotherapy, or hormone therapy, depending on the individual case. Advanced-stage breast cancer may require more aggressive treatment, such as chemotherapy, targeted therapy, or a combination of treatments.

*The various types of breast cancer.

There are several types of breast cancer, which can be classified based on the specific cells that are affected. The most common types of breast cancer are:

1. Ductal carcinoma: This is the most common type of breast cancer, accounting for about 80% of all cases. It begins in the cells that line the milk ducts in the breast.

2. Lobular carcinoma: This type of breast cancer begins in the cells that line the lobules, which are the milk-producing glands in the breast.

3. Inflammatory breast cancer: This is a rare and

aggressive form of breast cancer that causes the breast to become red, swollen, and tender.

4. Triple-negative breast cancer: This type of breast cancer is called "triple-negative" because it does not have receptors for estrogen, progesterone, or HER2/neu. It is more common in younger women and tends to be more aggressive than other types of breast cancer.

5. HER2-positive breast cancer: This type of breast cancer has too much of a protein called HER2/neu, which promotes the growth of cancer cells. It tends to be more aggressive than other types of breast cancer, but targeted therapies are available that can be effective in treating it.

6. Paget's disease of the nipple: This is a rare type of breast cancer that begins in the milk ducts and spreads to the skin of the nipple and areola. It can cause itching, redness, and scaling of the nipple and surrounding skin.

Treatment for breast cancer depends on the specific type of cancer and the stage of the disease. Treatment options may include surgery, radiation therapy, chemotherapy, hormone therapy, targeted therapy, or a combination of these approaches.

*The roles of genetics and environmental factors in the

development of breast cancer.

Breast cancer is a complex disease that results from a combination of genetic and environmental factors. While genetics can play a role in the development of breast cancer, the majority of breast cancer cases are not hereditary.

Genetic factors that increase the risk of breast cancer include mutations in the BRCA1 and BRCA2 genes, as well as mutations in other genes such as TP53, PTEN, and CHEK2. Women who inherit mutations in these genes have a significantly higher risk of developing breast cancer compared to women without the mutations.

Environmental factors that can increase the risk of breast cancer include lifestyle choices such as alcohol consumption, smoking, and lack of physical activity. Other environmental factors that may increase the risk of breast cancer include exposure to certain chemicals and radiation.

It's important to note that while these factors can increase the risk of breast cancer, having one or more risk factors does not necessarily mean that a woman will develop breast cancer. Additionally, some women with breast cancer may not have any known risk factors.

Regular mammograms and clinical breast exams are important for early detection of breast cancer. Women who have a family history of breast cancer or other risk factors may benefit from additional screening or risk-reducing measures such as prophylactic surgery or chemoprevention.

<u>Chapter 2.</u>

Causes and Risk Factors

In this chapter, we will explore the different causes of breast cancer, including genetic mutations, exposure to harmful chemicals, and lifestyle factors such as smoking and poor diet. We will also discuss the risk factors associated with breast cancer, such as age, family history, and certain medical conditions.

*Causes and risk factors of breast cancer.

Breast cancer is a complex disease, and its exact causes are not fully understood. However, several risk factors have been identified that can increase a woman's likelihood of developing breast cancer. Some of the main causes and risk factors of breast cancer include:

1. Age: The risk of breast cancer increases with age, especially after menopause.

2. Genetics: Women with mutations in certain genes, such as BRCA1 and BRCA2, have a higher risk of developing breast cancer.

3. Family history: A woman's risk of breast cancer is higher if she has a first-degree relative (mother, sister,

daughter) who has been diagnosed with breast cancer.

4. Hormonal factors: Long-term exposure to estrogen and progesterone, such as through hormone replacement therapy or starting menstruation at an early age, can increase the risk of breast cancer.

5. Lifestyle factors: Certain lifestyle factors, such as being overweight or obese, not getting enough physical activity, drinking alcohol, and smoking, can increase the risk of breast cancer.

6. Radiation exposure: Women who have undergone radiation therapy to the chest area for another medical condition, such as Hodgkin's lymphoma, have a higher risk of developing breast cancer.

It's important to note that having one or more of these risk factors does not necessarily mean that a woman will develop breast cancer. Many women who develop breast cancer have no known risk factors. Regular breast cancer screenings, including mammograms and clinical breast exams, are important for early detection and treatment of breast cancer.

Chapter 3.

Symptoms and Diagnosis

In this chapter, we will discuss the symptoms of breast cancer and how they vary depending on the type and stage of breast cancer. We will also explore the various diagnostic tests and procedures used to detect breast cancer, including mammograms, ultrasounds, MRIs, and biopsies.

*The Symptoms of breast cancer.

Breast cancer can present with a variety of symptoms, but not all women with breast cancer experience symptoms. It's important to note that some of these symptoms can also be caused by non-cancerous conditions. Regular breast cancer screenings, including mammograms and clinical breast exams, are important for early detection and treatment of breast cancer.

The symptoms of breast cancer can vary depending on the type and stage of the cancer. Some common symptoms of breast cancer include:

1. A lump or mass in the breast: This is the most common symptom of breast cancer, and it can feel like a hard, painless lump or a soft, tender lump.

2. Changes in the size or shape of the breast: Breast cancer can cause one breast to become larger or smaller than the other breast, or it can cause the breast to change shape.

3. Nipple discharge: A clear or bloody discharge from the nipple may be a sign of breast cancer.

4. Nipple inversion or retraction: A nipple that becomes inverted (pulled inward) or retracted (drawn back into the breast) may be a sign of breast cancer.

5. Skin changes: Breast cancer can cause changes to the skin of the breast, such as redness, thickening, or dimpling.

6. Breast pain: While breast cancer is not usually painful, some women may experience breast pain or discomfort.

The symptoms of breast cancer can also vary depending on the stage of the cancer. In the early stages, breast cancer may not cause any symptoms at all. As the cancer grows and spreads, it may cause more noticeable symptoms, such as:

1. Enlarged lymph nodes under the arm or in the collarbone area.

2. Swelling or lump in the chest or neck.

3. Shortness of breath or chest pain.

4. Bone pain or fractures (if the cancer has spread to the bones).

5. Loss of appetite or weight loss.

It's important to note that not all breast lumps are cancerous, and not all women with breast cancer will experience symptoms. If you notice any changes in your breasts, such as a lump or mass, changes in the size or shape of the breast, or nipple discharge, you should see a healthcare provider for an evaluation. Regular breast cancer screenings, including mammograms and clinical breast exams, are important for early detection and treatment of breast cancer.

*How to detect breast cancer.

There are several diagnostic tests and procedures used to detect breast cancer, including:

1. Mammogram: A mammogram is an X-ray of the breast that can detect early signs of breast cancer, such as a lump or mass.

2. Breast ultrasound: A breast ultrasound uses sound waves to create an image of the breast tissue and can help determine if a lump is a solid mass or a fluid-filled cyst.

3. Magnetic resonance imaging (MRI): An MRI uses a magnetic field and radio waves to create detailed images of the breast tissue. An MRI may be used in women with a high risk of breast cancer or to further evaluate suspicious findings on a mammogram or ultrasound.

4. Biopsy: A biopsy is a procedure in which a sample of breast tissue is removed and examined under a microscope to determine if cancer cells are present. There are several types of biopsies, including fine-needle aspiration, core-needle biopsy, and surgical biopsy.

5. Breast-specific gamma imaging (BSGI): BSGI is a nuclear medicine imaging technique that uses a radioactive tracer to detect breast cancer. It may be used in women with dense breast tissue or to further evaluate suspicious findings on a mammogram or ultrasound.

6. Breast duct endoscopy: A breast duct endoscopy is a minimally invasive procedure that allows a healthcare provider to examine the inside of the breast ducts using a thin, flexible tube with a camera on the end.

7. Molecular breast imaging (MBI): MBI is a nuclear medicine imaging technique that uses a radioactive tracer to detect breast cancer. It may be used in women with dense breast tissue or to further evaluate suspicious findings on a mammogram or ultrasound.

These tests and procedures can help detect breast cancer at an early stage when treatment is most effective. Women should talk to their healthcare provider about which tests are appropriate for their individual needs and risk factors.

<u>Chapter 4.</u>

Treatment Options

In this chapter, we will explore the different treatment options available for breast cancer, including surgery, radiation therapy, chemotherapy, immunotherapy, and targeted therapy. We will discuss the benefits and risks of each treatment and how they are selected based on the type and stage of breast cancer.

There are several treatment options available for breast cancer, and the best treatment plan will depend on the type and stage of the cancer, as well as the patient's overall health and personal preferences. The main treatments for breast cancer include:

*Treatment Options and their risks.

1. Surgery: Surgery is usually the first treatment for breast cancer and involves removing the cancerous tissue from the breast. There are different types of breast cancer surgery, including lumpectomy (removal of the tumor and surrounding tissue) and mastectomy (removal of the entire breast). The risks of surgery include bleeding, infection, and scarring.

2. Radiation therapy: Radiation therapy uses high-energy X

-rays to kill cancer cells and is often used after surgery to destroy any remaining cancer cells. The risks of radiation therapy include skin irritation and damage, fatigue, and long-term effects such as an increased risk of heart disease.

3. Chemotherapy: Chemotherapy uses drugs to kill cancer cells and is usually given after surgery to reduce the risk of the cancer returning. The risks of chemotherapy include nausea, hair loss, fatigue, and an increased risk of infection.

4. Hormone therapy: Hormone therapy is used to treat breast cancers that are hormone receptor-positive, meaning they grow in response to hormones such as estrogen. Hormone therapy blocks the effects of these hormones on the cancer cells or reduces the amount of hormones in the body. The risks of hormone therapy include hot flashes, fatigue, and an increased risk of osteoporosis.

5. Targeted therapy: Targeted therapy drugs specifically target cancer cells and can be used to treat HER2-positive breast cancers. The risks of targeted therapy include nausea, fatigue, and an increased risk of heart disease.

In addition to these treatments, there are also clinical trials testing new treatments for breast cancer. These trials can offer patients access to promising new treatments, but they also carry risks, including side effects and the possibility that the new treatment may not work.

The risks of each treatment depend on the individual patient and the specifics of their cancer. Patients should talk to their healthcare provider about the risks and benefits of each treatment option and how to manage any potential side effects.

<u>Chapter 5.</u>

Living with Breast Cancer

In this chapter, we will discuss the emotional and psychological impact of breast cancer on patients and their loved ones. We will explore strategies for coping with breast cancer, including support groups, counseling, and mindfulness practices. We will also discuss the importance of self-care and maintaining a healthy lifestyle during and after breast cancer treatment.

*The Emotional and Psychological impacts.

Breast cancer is a life-altering diagnosis that can have a significant emotional and psychological impact on both patients and their loved ones. Some of the common emotional and psychological responses to a breast cancer diagnosis include:

1. Fear and anxiety: Fear and anxiety are common responses to a cancer diagnosis. Patients may worry about their prognosis, treatment options, and the impact of the disease on their family and loved ones.

2. Depression: Breast cancer can cause depression in patients, who may feel sad, hopeless, or overwhelmed by the challenges of the disease.

3. Anger and frustration: Patients may feel angry or

frustrated at the diagnosis, the treatment process, or the impact of the disease on their lives.

4. Body image concerns: Breast cancer treatments can cause physical changes to the body, such as hair loss or mastectomy, which can impact a patient's self-esteem and body image.

5. Relationship strain: Breast cancer can also strain relationships, as patients may require significant emotional and practical support from their loved ones.

For loved ones, the emotional impact of breast cancer can be significant as well. They may experience fear, anxiety, and helplessness as they watch their loved one go through treatment. They may also experience caregiver burden, which can impact their own emotional well-being and quality of life.

It's important for patients and their loved ones to seek emotional and psychological support during and after breast cancer treatment. This may include talking to a therapist, joining a support group, or seeking out other resources to help cope with the emotional impact of the disease. By addressing the emotional and psychological impact of breast cancer, patients and their loved ones can improve their quality of life and overall well-being.

*Strategies for coping with breast cancer.

Coping with breast cancer can be challenging, but there are strategies that patients can use to help manage the emotional and physical effects of the disease. Here are some coping strategies that may be helpful:

1. Seek emotional support: Breast cancer can be an emotional rollercoaster, and it's important to have a support system in place. This may include talking to a therapist, joining a support group, or confiding in close friends and family members.

2. Take care of your physical health: A healthy diet, regular exercise, and getting enough rest can help patients cope with the physical effects of breast cancer treatment.

3. Learn about your diagnosis and treatment options: Educating yourself about breast cancer and the treatment options available can help you feel more in control and make informed decisions about your care.

4. Practice stress-reducing techniques: Techniques like deep breathing, meditation, and yoga can help reduce stress and promote relaxation.

5. Consider complementary therapies: Complementary therapies like acupuncture, massage, and aromatherapy

may help alleviate some of the physical and emotional symptoms of breast cancer treatment.

6. Focus on the present moment: Staying focused on the present moment and taking things one day at a time can help reduce anxiety and overwhelm.

7. Ask for help when you need it: Breast cancer treatment can be challenging, and it's okay to ask for help when you need it. This may include asking for help with household tasks, childcare, or transportation to appointments.

It's important for patients to find coping strategies that work for them and to be kind to themselves during the process. Coping with breast cancer is a journey, and it's important to take things one day at a time and celebrate small victories along the way.

*The importance of self-care and maintaining a healthy lifestyle during and after breast cancer treatment.

Self-care and maintaining a healthy lifestyle are important aspects of breast cancer treatment and recovery. Here's why:

1. Promotes physical health: A healthy lifestyle can help manage physical side effects of treatment, such as fatigue, pain, and nausea. Eating a healthy diet and engaging in

regular exercise can also help reduce the risk of recurrence and improve overall health.

2. Boosts emotional well-being: Self-care practices like meditation, yoga, and journaling can help reduce stress and improve emotional well-being. Taking care of oneself can also improve self-esteem and promote a positive body image.

3. Helps manage side effects: Self-care practices can also help manage side effects of treatment, such as anxiety, depression, and sleep disturbances.

4. Encourages self-advocacy: By prioritizing self-care, patients can learn to advocate for their own needs and take an active role in their treatment and recovery.

5. Promotes long-term health: A healthy lifestyle after breast cancer treatment can reduce the risk of other health conditions, such as heart disease, diabetes, and osteoporosis.

Some self-care practices that can be helpful during and after breast cancer treatment include:

1. Eating a healthy diet: A diet rich in fruits, vegetables, whole grains, and lean proteins can help manage side effects of treatment and improve overall health.

2. Engaging in regular exercise: Regular exercise can help

reduce fatigue, improve mood, and promote overall health. Patients should talk to their healthcare team before starting an exercise program.

3. Practicing stress-reducing techniques: Techniques like deep breathing, meditation, and yoga can help reduce stress and promote relaxation.

4. Getting enough sleep: Good sleep hygiene, such as avoiding screens before bed and creating a relaxing sleep environment, can help improve sleep quality.

5. Connecting with others: Maintaining social connections and seeking support from loved ones and support groups can improve emotional well-being and reduce feelings of isolation.

By prioritizing self-care and maintaining a healthy lifestyle, patients can improve their physical and emotional well-being during and after breast cancer treatment.

Chapter 6.

Breast Cancer Surgery

In this chapter, we will discuss the different types of breast cancer surgery, including lumpectomy, mastectomy, and breast reconstruction. We will explore the benefits and risks of each procedure and how they are selected based on the type and stage of breast cancer.

Breast cancer surgery is the most common treatment for breast cancer. There are several types of breast cancer surgery, including lumpectomy, mastectomy, and breast reconstruction. The type of surgery that a patient undergoes depends on the type and stage of breast cancer they have, as well as other factors such as the patient's age and overall health.

Lumpectomy:

A lumpectomy, also known as breast-conserving surgery, is a surgical procedure in which only the tumor and a small margin of surrounding breast tissue are removed. The goal of a lumpectomy is to remove the cancerous tissue while preserving as much of the breast tissue as possible. This procedure is usually recommended for patients with early-stage breast cancer where the tumor is small and confined to one area of the breast. Lumpectomy is often followed by radiation therapy to ensure that any remaining cancer cells are destroyed.

Benefits:

- Preservation of the breast tissue.

- Shorter recovery time and less discomfort compared to mastectomy.

- May be a better cosmetic outcome compared to mastectomy.

- Lower risk of complications such as infection or bleeding.

Risks:

- Possibility of cancer recurrence.

- Radiation therapy may cause skin changes or other side effects.

- Lumpectomy may not be an option if the tumor is too large or the cancer has spread throughout the breast tissue.

Mastectomy:

A mastectomy is a surgical procedure in which the entire breast is removed. This procedure is usually recommended for patients with larger tumors or for patients with multiple tumors in the same breast. In some cases, a mastectomy may be recommended as a preventive measure for patients at high risk of developing breast cancer.

Benefits:

- Removes the entire breast tissue, reducing the risk of cancer recurrence.

- May be the only option for patients with larger tumors or tumors in multiple areas of the breast.

- Breast reconstruction can be performed immediately or later on, depending on the patient's preference.

Risks:

- Longer recovery time and more discomfort compared to lumpectomy

- Possible complications such as infection or bleeding

- Cosmetic outcome may not be as good as lumpectomy followed by radiation therapy.

Breast Reconstruction:

Breast reconstruction is a surgical procedure that is performed to rebuild the breast after a mastectomy. There are several techniques for breast reconstruction, including breast implants or tissue flap procedures. Breast reconstruction can be performed at the same time as a mastectomy or at a later date.

Benefits:

- Restores the appearance of the breast.

- Can improve self-esteem and body image.

- Can be performed immediately after a mastectomy or at a later date.

Risks:

- Possible complications such as infection, bleeding, or implant rupture.

- Additional surgeries may be required.

- Longer recovery time compared to mastectomy alone.

In conclusion, the type of breast cancer surgery that a patient undergoes depends on several factors, including the type and stage of breast cancer, the patient's age and overall health, and the patient's preference. Lumpectomy, mastectomy, and breast reconstruction are all viable treatment options for breast cancer, and each option has its own benefits and risks. It is important for patients to discuss their options with their healthcare provider to

determine the best course of treatment for their individual
needs.

<u>Chapter 7.</u>

Radiation Therapy for Breast Cancer

In this chapter, we will discuss the role of radiation

therapy in breast cancer treatment, including the benefits and risks of this treatment. We will also explore the different types of radiation therapy and how they are used in breast cancer treatment.

Radiation therapy is a commonly used treatment for breast cancer, and it is often used in combination with surgery or chemotherapy. Radiation therapy uses high-energy radiation to destroy cancer cells or to prevent them from growing and dividing. The goal of radiation therapy in breast cancer treatment is to reduce the risk of cancer recurrence and to improve the patient's chances of survival.

Benefits of Radiation Therapy in Breast Cancer Treatment:

Radiation therapy offers several benefits in breast cancer treatment, including:

1. Reducing the risk of local recurrence: Radiation therapy can destroy any cancer cells that may remain in the breast after surgery, reducing the risk of local recurrence.

2. Increasing survival rates: Studies have shown that radiation therapy can improve survival rates in women

with breast cancer, particularly in those with larger tumors or cancer that has spread to the lymph nodes.

3. Minimizing the need for mastectomy: In some cases, radiation therapy can be used as an alternative to mastectomy, allowing women to preserve their breast.

Types of Radiation Therapy in Breast Cancer Treatment:

There are two main types of radiation therapy used in breast cancer treatment: external beam radiation therapy and brachytherapy.

1. External beam radiation therapy: This type of radiation therapy uses a machine that delivers high-energy radiation beams to the breast from outside the body. The radiation is targeted to the breast tissue and surrounding lymph nodes.

2. Brachytherapy: This type of radiation therapy involves placing small radioactive seeds or sources directly into the breast tissue. The radiation is delivered from inside the body and targets the area surrounding the tumor.

Risks of Radiation Therapy in Breast Cancer Treatment:

Radiation therapy does come with some risks, including:

1. Skin irritation: Radiation therapy can cause skin irritation, redness, and dryness in the treated area.

2. Fatigue: Radiation therapy can cause fatigue and tiredness, particularly towards the end of the treatment course.

3. Lymphedema: Radiation therapy can cause swelling in the arm and hand on the side of the breast where treatment was given, particularly in women who have also had lymph nodes removed.

4. Rare long-term risks: In rare cases, radiation therapy can increase the risk of developing another cancer in the treated area, although this risk is generally small.

Overall, radiation therapy is an effective treatment option for many women with breast cancer. The benefits of radiation therapy generally outweigh the risks, and the type of radiation therapy used will depend on the individual case and the extent of the cancer.

Chapter 8.

Chemotherapy for Breast Cancer

In this chapter, we will discuss the role of chemotherapy in breast cancer treatment, including the benefits and risks of this treatment. We will also explore the different types of chemotherapy and how they are used in breast cancer treatment.

Chemotherapy is one of the main treatments for breast cancer, which involves the use of drugs to kill cancer cells throughout the body. In this response, I will discuss the role of chemotherapy in breast cancer treatment, including the benefits and risks of this treatment, as well as the different types of chemotherapy and how they are used in breast cancer treatment.

Role of Chemotherapy in Breast Cancer Treatment:

Chemotherapy is often used in breast cancer treatment to destroy cancer cells that may have spread beyond the breast or lymph nodes. The use of chemotherapy depends on the stage of the breast cancer, the size of the tumor, and other factors such as hormone receptor status, HER2 status, and age of the patient. Chemotherapy is often used after surgery (adjuvant chemotherapy) to reduce the risk of cancer recurrence or before surgery (neoadjuvant chemotherapy) to shrink the tumor and make it easier to remove.

Benefits of Chemotherapy:

Chemotherapy can be very effective in killing cancer cells and reducing the risk of cancer recurrence. It may also shrink the tumor, making it easier to remove with surgery. In addition, chemotherapy can help control symptoms and improve quality of life for patients with advanced breast cancer.

Risks of Chemotherapy:

Chemotherapy can cause a number of side effects, including hair loss, nausea, vomiting, fatigue, and an increased risk of infection. In addition, chemotherapy can affect healthy cells in the body, leading to long-term side effects such as heart damage, nerve damage, and an increased risk of leukemia.

Types of Chemotherapy:

There are several types of chemotherapy drugs used in breast cancer treatment, including anthracyclines, taxanes, antimetabolites, and platinum drugs. Anthracyclines, such as doxorubicin and epirubicin, are often used in combination with other drugs and can be effective in treating early-stage and advanced breast cancer. Taxanes, such as paclitaxel and docetaxel, are often used in combination with anthracyclines and are effective in treating early-stage and advanced breast cancer. Antimetabolites, such as capecitabine and methotrexate, work by blocking the enzymes that cancer cells need to grow and divide. Platinum drugs, such as cisplatin and carboplatin, can also be used in breast cancer treatment and work by interfering with DNA synthesis in cancer cells.

In conclusion, chemotherapy is an important treatment option for breast cancer and can be very effective in reducing the risk of cancer recurrence. However, it can also cause a number of side effects and long-term risks. The type of chemotherapy used depends on the stage and characteristics of the breast cancer, and it is usually given in combination with other treatments such as surgery, radiation therapy, and targeted therapy.

Chapter 9.

Hormone Therapy for Breast Cancer

In this chapter, we will discuss the role of hormone therapy in breast cancer treatment, including the benefits and risks of this treatment. We will also explore the different types of hormone therapy and how they are used in breast cancer treatment.

Hormone therapy is a common treatment for breast cancer that is hormone receptor-positive. This type of breast cancer grows in response to hormones, such as estrogen or progesterone. In this response, I will discuss the role of hormone therapy in breast cancer treatment, including the benefits and risks of this treatment, as well as the different types of hormone therapy and how they are used in breast cancer treatment.

Role of Hormone Therapy in Breast Cancer Treatment:

Hormone therapy works by blocking the effects of hormones, such as estrogen or progesterone, on cancer cells. This can slow or stop the growth of hormone receptor-positive breast cancer. Hormone therapy is often used after surgery (adjuvant therapy) to reduce the risk of cancer recurrence or to treat advanced breast cancer.

Benefits of Hormone Therapy:

Hormone therapy can be very effective in treating hormone receptor-positive breast cancer. It can reduce the risk of cancer recurrence and improve survival rates. In addition, hormone therapy often has fewer side effects than other breast cancer treatments, such as chemotherapy.

Risks of Hormone Therapy:

Hormone therapy can cause a number of side effects, including hot flashes, vaginal dryness, mood changes, and an increased risk of blood clots or stroke. In addition, long-term use of hormone therapy can increase the risk of osteoporosis and bone fractures.

Types of Hormone Therapy:

There are several types of hormone therapy used in breast cancer treatment, including:

- Tamoxifen: This is a type of selective estrogen receptor modulator (SERM) that blocks the effects of estrogen on cancer cells. It is often used to treat both early-stage and advanced breast cancer.

- Aromatase inhibitors: These drugs block the production

of estrogen in postmenopausal women, as the ovaries stop producing estrogen at this time. Aromatase inhibitors are often used after surgery to reduce the risk of cancer recurrence.

- **Fulvestrant:** This is a type of selective estrogen receptor degrader (SERD) that binds to and destroys estrogen receptors on cancer cells, making them unable to respond to estrogen. It is often used to treat advanced breast cancer.

In conclusion, hormone therapy is an important treatment option for hormone receptor-positive breast cancer. It works by blocking the effects of hormones on cancer cells, slowing or stopping their growth. Hormone therapy has several types, including tamoxifen, aromatase inhibitors, and fulvestrant, and they are often used after surgery to reduce the risk of cancer recurrence or to treat advanced breast cancer. Hormone therapy has benefits, but also side effects, and women should discuss the risks and benefits of hormone therapy with their healthcare provider to determine the best treatment plan for them.

Chapter 10.

Targeted Therapy for Breast Cancer

In this chapter, we will discuss the role of targeted therapy in breast cancer treatment, including the benefits and risks of this treatment. We will also explore the different types of targeted therapy and how they are used in breast cancer treatment.

Targeted therapy is a type of cancer treatment that targets specific molecules involved in the growth and spread of cancer cells. In breast cancer, targeted therapy is often used in combination with other treatments, such as chemotherapy or hormone therapy, to treat advanced or metastatic breast cancer. In this response, I will discuss the role of targeted therapy in breast cancer treatment, including the benefits and risks of this treatment, as well as the different types of targeted therapy and how they are used in breast cancer treatment.

Role of Targeted Therapy in Breast Cancer Treatment:

Targeted therapy is designed to specifically target cancer cells while sparing healthy cells. It works by targeting molecules or pathways that are involved in the growth and spread of cancer cells. Targeted therapy can be used to treat different types of breast cancer, including HER2-positive breast cancer and triple-negative breast cancer.

Benefits of Targeted Therapy:

Targeted therapy can be very effective in treating breast cancer, especially in cases where other treatments, such as chemotherapy, have not been effective. It can improve survival rates and reduce the risk of cancer recurrence. In addition, targeted therapy often has fewer side effects than other cancer treatments, such as chemotherapy.

Risks of Targeted Therapy:

Targeted therapy can cause a number of side effects, including fatigue, nausea, diarrhea, and skin rash. In addition, some targeted therapies can affect the heart and liver, and may cause changes in blood pressure, heart rate, or other cardiac parameters. Targeted therapy can also be expensive and may not be covered by all insurance plans.

Types of Targeted Therapy:

There are several types of targeted therapy used in breast

cancer treatment, including:

- **HER2-targeted therapy**: HER2 is a protein that is overexpressed in about 20% of breast cancers. HER2-targeted therapy works by targeting the HER2 protein, which slows or stops the growth of HER2-positive breast cancer cells. Examples of HER2-targeted therapy include trastuzumab, pertuzumab, and ado-trastuzumab emtansine (T-DM1).

- **CDK4/6 inhibitors**: Cyclin-dependent kinase (CDK) 4/6 inhibitors work by blocking proteins that help cancer cells divide and grow. They are used in combination with hormone therapy to treat hormone receptor-positive breast cancer. Examples of CDK4/6 inhibitors include palbociclib, ribociclib, and abemaciclib.

- **PARP inhibitors**: Poly (ADP-ribose) polymerase (PARP) inhibitors work by blocking a protein that helps repair damaged DNA in cancer cells. They are used to treat triple-negative breast cancer and certain other breast cancers that have a BRCA gene mutation. Examples of PARP inhibitors include olaparib, talazoparib, and rucaparib.

In conclusion, targeted therapy is an important treatment option for breast cancer, especially for HER2-positive and triple-negative breast cancer. It works by targeting specific molecules involved in the growth and spread of cancer cells. Targeted therapy has benefits, but also side effects, and women should discuss the risks and benefits of targeted therapy with their healthcare provider to determine the best treatment plan for them.

<u>Chapter 11.</u>

Breast Cancer Prevention

In this chapter, we will explore strategies for preventing breast cancer, including lifestyle changes, early detection, and genetic testing. We will discuss the importance of breast self-exams, mammograms, and other screening tests for breast cancer.

Breast cancer is one of the most common types of cancer in women, but there are strategies that can help reduce the risk of developing breast cancer. In this response, I will discuss various strategies for preventing breast cancer, including lifestyle changes, early detection, and genetic testing. I will also discuss the importance of breast self-exams, mammograms, and other screening tests for breast cancer.

1. Lifestyle Changes:

Making certain lifestyle changes can help reduce the risk of breast cancer. These include:

- Maintaining a healthy weight

- Eating a balanced diet with plenty of fruits and vegetables

- Exercising regularly

- Limiting alcohol intake

- Avoiding smoking and second-hand smoke

- Limiting exposure to environmental toxins

2. Early Detection:

Early detection is key to treating breast cancer successfully. Regular screenings can help detect breast cancer in its early stages, making it easier to treat. Women should be aware of the following screening tests:

- Breast self-exams: Women should perform regular breast self-exams to detect any changes in their breasts.

- Mammograms: Women aged 50-74 should have a mammogram every two years. Women with a family history of breast cancer may need to start screening earlier or have more frequent screenings.

- Clinical breast exams: Women should have a clinical breast exam by a healthcare professional at least every three years.

3. Genetic Testing:

Women with a family history of breast cancer may be at higher risk of developing the disease. Genetic testing can help determine if a woman has inherited a gene mutation that increases her risk of breast cancer. If a woman is found to have a gene mutation, she may be advised to have more frequent screenings or take preventive measures such as a prophylactic mastectomy.

In conclusion, breast cancer prevention involves making certain lifestyle changes, early detection through regular screenings, and genetic testing for women with a family history of breast cancer. Breast self-exams, mammograms, and clinical breast exams are important screening tests for detecting breast cancer in its early stages. Women should speak to their healthcare provider about their risk of developing breast cancer and develop a personalized plan for breast cancer prevention and screening.